COMPLETE GUIDE TO PANCREATITIS

A Comprehensive Handbook For Understanding, Managing, Healing, Nutritional Strategies, Holistic Approaches For Rapid Recovery And Long-Term Wellness

DEHART HAIRSTON

DISCLAIMER

This book's content is only intended for general informative purposes. At the time of writing, the author has taken every precaution to guarantee that the material is correct and current. Nevertheless, the author disclaims all explicit and implicit representations and guarantees about the availability, appropriateness, correctness, completeness, and usefulness of the material on these pages.

Since the author is not a licensed medical practitioner, the material in this book shouldn't be interpreted as medical advice. Before making any modifications to their diet, exercise regimen, or medical treatment, readers are urged to speak with a licensed healthcare provider.

Moreover, the author has no connection to any of the businesses, organizations, or people that are discussed in this book. Any mentions of goods, services, businesses, or people are purely informative and do not indicate endorsement or suggestion.

This book's content is entirely dependent on the author's expertise, study, and comprehension of the topic. Despite having taken reasonable care to offer correct information, the author disclaims all liability for any mistakes or omissions in the material as well as for any losses, harm, or damages resulting from using the information.

It is recommended that readers use their own judgment and discretion when applying the knowledge in this book to their own situations. The use or implementation of any material in this book may result in unfavorable repercussions, directly or indirectly, for which the author assumes no liability.

By reading this book, you agree to release and hold the author harmless from any claims, losses, liabilities, costs, or expenditures resulting from or related to the use of the information you get from it.

Table of Contents

ABOUT THE BOOK

"Pancreatitis" is a detailed handbook that may be a lifesaver for anybody afflicted with this ailment; it is not simply another medical book. It is important to comprehend the complexities of pancreatitis, and this book explores all of its facets. Chapter 1 provides readers with an overview of the disease, including its definition, causes, and kinds.

Going forward, Chapter 2 offers a priceless insight into the pancreas's architecture, functioning, and the reasons why keeping it healthy is crucial. With this information, it becomes simpler to recognize the symptoms and indicators (Chapter 3), enabling readers to comprehend the possible consequences linked to the illness and when to seek medical attention.

Making an accurate diagnosis of pancreatitis (Chapter 4) is often the first step toward appropriate management. This book explains the various medical tests, making it easier for readers to understand their findings and emphasizing the value of early detection.

Further treatment options, including as drugs, dietary modifications, and surgical procedures, are covered in Chapter 5. In Chapter 6, the compassionate care of pancreatitis pain is discussed, along with coping mechanisms, pain relief methods, and complementary therapies.

However, this book goes beyond only treating pancreatic disease; Chapter 7, highlights the significance of lifestyle modifications, covering everything from quitting smoking and drinking to embracing exercise and stress reduction. Another major emphasis is prevention (Chapter 8), where readers may protect themselves from pancreatitis by following the suggested healthy behaviors and useful advice.

It may be difficult to live with pancreatitis (Chapter 9), but this book helps readers preserve their quality of life by providing tools, support networks, and information on the psychological effects. In Chapter 10, the book concludes by discussing future directions in research, treatment options, and advocacy initiatives, all of which inspire optimism and drive.

"Pancreatitis" is essentially a must-have resource for everyone affected by this illness, providing not just knowledge but also empowerment, support, and a path to improved health and wellness.

CHAPTER 1

Understanding Pancreatitis

What Is Pancreatitis?

The symptoms of pancreatitis, a disorder marked by pancreatic inflammation, may vary from little pain to a serious, perhaps fatal sickness. The pancreas, which is situated beneath the stomach, produces hormones and enzymes like insulin that are essential for digestion and blood sugar management. Inflammation of the pancreas may result in several symptoms and problems.

When the pancreatic digestion enzymes are engaged while the organ is still within, pancreatic tissue is harmed, leading to pancreatitis and inflammation. Several conditions, including gallstones, infections, alcoholism, and certain drugs, may cause this activation.

It is crucial to comprehend the signs and risk factors of pancreatitis to diagnose and treat the condition promptly.

Causes Of Pancreatitis

Numerous factors, from medical issues to lifestyle choices, may induce pancreatitis. The most frequent reason is overindulgence in alcohol. Prolonged heavy alcohol use may cause the pancreas to become irritated and inflamed, which can result in pancreatitis. Gallstones are another typical reason; they may obstruct the pancreatic duct, preventing the passage of digestive enzymes, which build up and cause inflammation.

Several treatments, including immunosuppressants, chemotherapeutic agents, and certain antibiotics, may potentially raise the risk of pancreatitis by directly irritating or impairing the pancreas. Pancreatic inflammation may also result from infections, including bacterial or viral infections. Furthermore, pancreatitis may result from raised blood triglyceride levels, which are a kind of fat.

It is essential to comprehend the many causes of pancreatitis to avoid and treat the condition. To relieve symptoms and stop recurrence, healthcare professionals may create a suitable treatment plan by identifying and treating the underlying cause.

Types Of Pancreatitis

Acute pancreatitis and chronic pancreatitis are the two primary forms of pancreatitis. Acute pancreatitis is the term for an abrupt beginning of pancreatic inflammation that, with the right care, usually goes away in a few days. Severe stomach pain, nausea, vomiting, and fever are typical signs of acute pancreatitis.

On the other hand, chronic pancreatitis is characterized by persistent and sometimes worsening pancreatic inflammation. Chronic pancreatitis may result in long-term problems such as pancreatic insufficiency, diabetes, and pancreatic cancer, in contrast to acute pancreatitis, which often goes away quickly. Recurrent stomach discomfort, diarrhea, weight loss, and steatorrhea (fatty stools) are some of the signs and symptoms of chronic pancreatitis.

Diagnosis and treatment of acute and chronic pancreatitis depend on an understanding of their distinctions. Acute pancreatitis often calls for hospitalization and supportive care, but long-term care may be necessary for chronic pancreatitis to manage symptoms and avoid complications. The kind of pancreatitis and its underlying causes may be determined, allowing medical professionals to customize treatment regimens to each patient's requirements.

CHAPTER 2

Anatomy Of The Pancreas

Introduction To The Pancreas

The pancreas, also called the "hidden organ" because of its unseen position, is essential to keeping our bodies balanced. Tucked away in the upper belly, this special organ performs both exocrine and endocrine duties. It is located behind the stomach. The exocrine component includes creating digestive enzymes necessary for meal digestion, while the endocrine component involves hormones sent directly into the circulation to control blood sugar levels.

The pancreas has a dual role in digestion and metabolism, which emphasizes its importance. Despite being smaller than other essential organs, it has a huge influence on general health. It is essential to appreciate the structure and functioning of the pancreas to successfully manage pancreatic health and to understand disorders such as pancreatitis.

Functions Of The Pancreas

The pancreas coordinates a symphony of processes essential to human health:

1. Endocrine Function: The release of hormones that control blood sugar levels, such as glucagon and insulin, is one of its main functions. After a meal, insulin helps cells absorb glucose from the circulation, decreasing blood sugar levels; when blood sugar levels fall too low, glucagon boosts them to provide a steady source of energy for the body.

2. Exocrine Function: The pancreas produces digestive enzymes that are essential for the breakdown of proteins, lipids, and carbohydrates in the digestive system, such as lipase, amylase, and

proteases. Enzymes aid in the process of absorbing nutrients from meals, maintaining body processes, and supplying energy.

3. **Production of Bicarbonate:** The pancreas secretes bicarbonate, an alkaline material that balances stomach acid as food passes through to the small intestine, in addition to enzymes. By neutralizing the acidic pH, this process preserves the vulnerable intestinal lining and fosters the ideal conditions for enzyme activation.

Importance Of Pancreatic Health

Sustaining ideal pancreas health is essential for general health:

1. **Digestive Efficiency:** Malnutrition and digestive diseases are avoided when the pancreas is in good condition since this guarantees effective digestion and nutrient absorption. Nutrient absorption is hampered when pancreatic function is impaired, as

in pancreatitis, which results in deficiencies and gastrointestinal symptoms such as bloating, diarrhea, and stomach discomfort.

2. Blood Sugar Regulation: To keep blood sugar levels steady, the pancreas must operate properly. In diabetes mellitus, disruptions in insulin synthesis or activity may lead to hyperglycemia (high blood sugar) or hypoglycemia (low blood sugar), both of which have significant health hazards if left unchecked.

3. General Health: The pancreas affects several body processes in addition to digestion and metabolism. To preserve homeostasis, it communicates with several organs and systems, including the liver, gallbladder, and endocrine glands. As a result, pancreatic illnesses may affect many aspects of health, including hormone balance, metabolism, immunity, and digestion.

Knowledge of the pancreas' complex structure and activities highlights the organ's critical role in health maintenance and emphasizes the need to take preventative action to protect it. People may prevent pancreatic problems and maximize their overall health and vitality by adopting healthy lifestyle practices such as frequent exercise, a balanced diet, and abstaining from excessive alcohol intake.

CHAPTER 3

Signs And Symptoms

Recognizing Symptoms Of Pancreatitis

The symptoms of pancreatitis may range from a little discomfort to excruciating agony. It is essential to comprehend these signs to diagnose and treat patients on time.

Abdominal discomfort, usually centered in the upper abdomen but sometimes extending to the back, is one of the most prevalent indicators of pancreatitis. This discomfort is usually worse after eating or drinking, and it may be dull and moderate or severe and chronic. Vomiting and nausea are also frequent because pancreatic inflammation impairs digestion and may cause gastrointestinal pain.

Pancreatitis may also cause fever, a fast heartbeat, and an overall sense of being unwell.

When inflammation reaches the bile ducts, it may result in jaundice, which is characterized by yellowing of the skin and eyes. Shock symptoms like fast breathing and low blood pressure may appear in extreme situations.

It's crucial to remember that each person's experience with pancreatitis will be unique in terms of the degree and mix of symptoms, as well as the underlying reason. Thus, early medical response depends on paying attention to any odd or persistent symptoms.

When To Seek Medical Help

It's critical to recognize when to seek medical attention for pancreatitis symptoms to avoid complications and guarantee proper treatment. While minor symptoms could go away on their own, serious or persistent symptoms need to be treated by a doctor right away.

It's imperative that you get medical attention right away if you have severe abdominal discomfort that doesn't go away or becomes worse over time. Likewise, it is important to pay attention to prolonged nausea, vomiting, and fever, particularly if they are accompanied by additional symptoms like jaundice or a fast pulse.

Certain warning indicators, such as extreme dehydration, fainting, or bewilderment, point to a potentially fatal circumstance. For immediate assessment and treatment in such circumstances, do not hesitate to contact emergency services or go to the closest emergency facility.

Furthermore, it's critical to pay close attention to any new or worsening symptoms if you have a history of pancreatitis or other risk factors like gallstones or alcohol addiction. Seeing a doctor regularly might help you stay on top of your health and avoid problems.

In the end, when it comes to pancreatitis symptoms, it's better to err on the side of caution. Early intervention and treatment are made possible by prompt medical examination, which enhances results and lowers the possibility of major problems.

Complications Associated With Pancreatitis

If ignored or improperly managed, pancreatitis may result in several complications that carry serious health concerns. To avoid long-term effects, individuals and healthcare professionals must both be aware of potential problems.

Pancreatic pseudocysts, which are fluid-filled sacs that form in or around the pancreas as a result of inflammation and tissue damage, are a typical consequence of pancreatitis. If these cysts get larger or become infected, they may need to be surgically removed or drained, which may result in nausea, vomiting, and abdominal discomfort.

Diabetes mellitus, malnourishment, and digestive issues may result from chronic pancreatitis, which is characterized by persistent inflammation and scarring of the pancreas. Weight loss and nutritional malabsorption may result from the pancreas' inability to generate enough enzymes to adequately digest food, a condition known as pancreatic insufficiency that can develop from chronic pancreatitis over time.

In extreme circumstances, acute pancreatitis may also result in systemic consequences such as organ failure, sepsis, and respiratory distress syndrome. To properly treat these potentially fatal consequences, medical intervention and intense care are necessary.

Furthermore, having recurrent bouts of pancreatitis raises the chance of getting pancreatic cancer, particularly in those who already have underlying risk factors including obesity, smoking, or genetic susceptibility. As a result, prompt pancreatitis diagnosis and treatment are essential for reducing symptoms, averting complications, and enhancing long-term results.

Patients and medical professionals may collaborate to take preventative steps, enhance treatment plans, and enhance overall patient care and quality of life by being aware of the possible consequences linked to pancreatitis.

CHAPTER 4

Diagnosing Pancreatitis

Medical Tests For Pancreatitis

Medical tests are essential in the diagnosis of pancreatitis since they help to explain the symptoms. These tests are intended to identify anomalies in the pancreas, assisting medical practitioners in correctly diagnosing the illness and formulating a treatment strategy.

Blood testing is one of the main methods used to diagnose pancreatitis. These tests measure the blood's concentrations of pancreatic enzymes like lipase and amylase. These enzymes' elevated levels often signify pancreatic inflammation. Furthermore, as pancreatitis sometimes impairs liver function, testing for liver health may also be performed.

Imaging examinations are another vital diagnostic tool. These consist of MRIs, CT scans, and ultrasounds. Utilizing sound waves, ultrasound produces pictures of the pancreas and its surrounding organs, offering important information about any inflammation or anomalies. CT scans may identify issues like fluid accumulations or abscesses and provide more comprehensive pictures. Pancreatitis and its consequences may be diagnosed more accurately with the use of magnetic fields and radio waves, which provide high-resolution pictures.

Endoscopic testing could be carried out under certain circumstances. To study the pancreas and bile ducts, endoscopic retrograde cholangiopancreatography (ERCP) entails passing a flexible tube equipped with a camera through the mouth and into the digestive system.

This process may assist in locating obstructions or other problems that may be causing pancreatitis.

Understanding Test Results

Understanding several characteristics and signs in a nuanced way is necessary when interpreting test results for pancreatitis. An indication of pancreatic inflammation is usually elevated levels of pancreatic enzymes, such as lipase and amylase. But it's important to take into account other variables, such as renal function and medication, which might affect these levels.

Visual confirmation of pancreatic abnormalities is provided by imaging testing. Pancreatic edema or fluid buildup may be seen using ultrasounds, but comprehensive pictures provided by CT and MRI scans can assist in determining the exact nature and degree of inflammation. To distinguish between pathogenic alterations linked to pancreatitis and normal variations, the interpretation of these pictures calls for specialized knowledge.

Endoscopic procedures like ERCPs may shed light on the underlying causes of pancreatitis. Finding tumors, strictures, or gallstones within the bile ducts or pancreas may assist guide treatment choices and stop recurring pancreatitis attacks.

Comprehending test data necessitates placing findings into the larger clinical context, going beyond just analyzing statistics or pictures. To establish an accurate diagnosis and create a successful treatment plan, medical experts must take into account the patient's symptoms, past medical history, and other test results.

Importance Of Early Diagnosis

For several reasons, a pancreatitis diagnosis made early is essential. First of all, it makes it possible to start treatment right away, which may help to reduce symptoms and avoid consequences. A delayed diagnosis may exacerbate inflammation, resulting in more severe symptoms and a higher chance of consequences including infection or pancreatic necrosis.

Moreover, quick identification and management of pancreatitis' underlying causes is made possible by early diagnosis by healthcare professionals. Determining the underlying cause of pancreatitis caused by medicine, alcoholism, or gallstones is crucial for averting recurrence and directing long-term treatment plans.

By lowering the chance of complications and decreasing the need for intrusive procedures, early diagnosis also improves patient outcomes. Acute necrotizing pancreatitis and chronic pancreatitis, which have greater rates of morbidity and death, are examples of more severe types of pancreatitis that may be avoided with prompt care.

Early diagnosis also makes it possible to put supportive measures like pain relief, dietary assistance, and problem monitoring into action quickly. These therapies have the potential to enhance the patient's quality of life and expedite their recuperation.

It is critical to diagnose pancreatitis as soon as possible to address underlying causes, start treatment on time, and avoid complications. To guarantee the best possible results for their patients, medical personnel need to be on the lookout for pancreatitis symptoms and indications and act quickly to order diagnostic tests when necessary.

CHAPTER 5

Treatment Options

Medications For Pancreatitis

Medication is a vital part of pancreatitis management since it helps to reduce symptoms and encourage recovery. Medication's main goals are to treat the condition's underlying causes or consequences, as well as to lessen inflammation and alleviate discomfort.

Painkillers are among the drugs that are often provided for pancreatitis. These may include heavier prescription drugs like opioids and over-the-counter alternatives like acetaminophen. Treatment for pancreatitis must include pain control since patients may have severe, incapacitating stomach discomfort due to pancreatic inflammation.

Enzyme supplements are another family of drugs that are often administered for pancreatitis. Pancreatic enzyme supplements are used to help with digesting since pancreatitis may disrupt the normal synthesis of digestive enzymes. By aiding in the body's breakdown of proteins, lipids, and carbs, these supplements enhance nutritional absorption and lessen the burden on the pancreas.

If gallstones are the cause of pancreatitis, prescription drugs may be needed to dissolve the stones. By gradually dissolving cholesterol-based gallstones, these drugs stop further pancreatic duct obstructions and lower the likelihood of repeated pancreatitis episodes.

If there are signs of infection in the pancreas or adjacent tissues, people with pancreatitis may also be offered antibiotics in addition to these drugs. Antibiotics aid in the fight against bacterial infections and guard against consequences like the development of an abscess or a systemic infection.

Dietary Changes And Nutrition Tips

Making dietary adjustments is essential for controlling pancreatitis and avoiding flare-ups. Given the critical function the pancreas plays in digestion, it is essential to follow a diet that is both high in nutrients and easy on the digestive tract.

Eating a low-fat diet is one of the main dietary suggestions for pancreatitis. Reducing fat consumption may help alleviate symptoms and lessen the strain on the pancreas since fat can cause the release of pancreatic enzymes and aggravate inflammation. meals heavy in trans and saturated fats, such as processed snacks, fatty meats, and fried meals, should be consumed in moderation or never.

Rather, concentrate on increasing your intake of whole grains, lean meats, fruits, and veggies. These meals are rich in vital nutrients and antioxidants that promote general health and healing, in addition to being reduced in fat.

Eating smaller, more frequent meals throughout the day is also helpful, as opposed to larger ones. This may lessen the chance of causing symptoms by preventing the pancreas from being overloaded with food all at once.

Dietary supplements could be advised in certain circumstances to guarantee sufficient nutritional intake, particularly if there are shortages brought on by malabsorption or poor digestion. To promote optimum nutrition and facilitate digestion, these supplements may include vitamins, minerals, and digestive enzymes.

Another important part of managing pancreatitis is staying hydrated. Water consumption promotes healthy hydration, aids in digestion, and removes toxins from the body. But because alcohol and sugar-filled drinks may aggravate inflammation and irritate the pancreas, it's crucial to stay away from them.

Surgical Interventions

Surgical surgery may be required in situations of severe or chronic pancreatitis that do not respond to conservative therapy techniques. The goals of pancreatitis surgery are to enhance the patient's quality of life by addressing complications, removing blockages, and relieving symptoms.

The Whipple surgery, also known as pancreaticoduodenectomy, is a frequent surgical treatment for pancreatitis. During this procedure, the duodenum, a section of the bile duct, the head of the pancreas, and sometimes the stomach are removed. When pancreatic cancer or severe chronic pancreatitis with consequences like blockages or pseudocysts occur, it is often done.

Drainage operations are another surgical option for pancreatitis. These operations may be carried out to remove fluid accumulations or pseudocysts that have developed within or outside of the pancreas. Drainage may lessen the chance of problems like infection or rupture while also helping to relieve symptoms like discomfort and pain in the abdomen.

In some instances, surgical intervention could be required to remove gallstones or treat anatomical anomalies in the bile or pancreatic ducts that are causing pancreatitis. The goals of these treatments are to stop inflammatory events from happening again and to return pancreatic function to normal.

Generally, when conservative measures have failed to relieve pancreatitis, surgery is only considered when the advantages of the procedure exceed the dangers. To choose the best course of action for their unique situation and medical history, individuals must go through all of their choices with their healthcare professionals.

CHAPTER 6

Managing Pain

Coping Strategies For Pancreatic Pain

Pancreatic discomfort may cause great suffering and affect not only one's physical health but also one's mental and emotional state of mind. Effective coping mechanisms are essential for handling this discomfort. Education is one of the most important coping mechanisms. Knowing the causes, characteristics, and physiological effects of pancreatic pain might help people better control their symptoms.

Creating a robust support system is a crucial coping tactic. Having compassionate friends, family, and medical experts around oneself may be a huge help when it comes to emotional support during trying times.

Joining online forums or support groups with others who have gone through similar things may also foster understanding and a feeling of togetherness.

Pancreatic discomfort may also be lessened by engaging in relaxation practices like yoga, meditation, or deep breathing. These methods lower stress levels, which may worsen pain, in addition to encouraging physical relaxation. Relieving oneself by focusing on fun pursuits, hobbies, or diversion from the discomfort might also help.

In addition, leading a healthy lifestyle that includes consistent exercise, a balanced diet, and enough water will improve general well-being and perhaps lessen the frequency and severity of pancreatic pain episodes. Collaborating closely with medical providers is crucial in creating a customized pain management strategy based on each patient's requirements and preferences.

Pain Management Techniques

Pancreatic pain treatment calls for a multimodal strategy that may include several pain relief methods. Medication is one of the main strategies for treating pain. To ease discomfort, doctors may give acetaminophen, nonsteroidal anti-inflammatory medications (NSAIDs), or prescription painkillers. To prevent any possible negative effects or difficulties, these drugs must be used under the supervision of a healthcare provider.

In rare circumstances, it could be advised to target certain nerves that the pancreas uses to relay pain signals by nerve blocks or neurolytic operations. For those who suffer from severe or persistent pancreatic discomfort, these treatments may provide either short-term or long-term relief.

Furthermore, some people may find relief with complementary treatments including massage therapy, acupuncture, or transcutaneous electrical nerve stimulation (TENS). These treatments function by encouraging relaxation, which may lessen the perception of pain, or by igniting the body's natural pain-relieving processes.

For the treatment of pancreatic pain, psychological therapies such as cognitive-behavioral therapy (CBT) may potentially be helpful. Even for those who experience chronic pain, cognitive behavioral therapy (CBT) may help them overcome negative thinking patterns, create coping mechanisms, and enhance their general quality of life.

It's important to experiment with different pain management strategies to see which ones each person responds to the best. To successfully control pancreatic pain and enhance quality of life, a variety of strategies, including medication, interventional procedures, alternative therapies, and psychological support, may be required.

Alternative Therapies

Alternative therapies may be used in conjunction with traditional medical treatments to help manage pancreatic discomfort. One such treatment is acupuncture, an old Chinese method of stimulating energy flow and promoting healing by putting tiny needles into certain body sites. Acupuncture is beneficial for certain people in terms of pain relief and general well-being.

Another complementary treatment that may help with pancreatic discomfort is massage therapy. Massage treatment can lessen stress, enhance circulation, and ease pancreatitis-related pain by exerting pressure on soft tissues and muscles.

Nutritional supplements and herbal therapies could provide further assistance in the management of pancreatic discomfort. For instance, the anti-inflammatory qualities of ginger and turmeric are well-known, and they may aid in lowering pancreatic inflammation. But before taking any herbal cures or supplements, it's important to speak with a doctor since they can worsen pre-existing problems or interfere with medicine.

For those with pancreatic discomfort, mind-body techniques like yoga, tai chi, or mindfulness meditation may also be helpful. These techniques encourage body awareness, relaxation, and stress reduction, all of which may help people manage their pain and live better overall.

Before implementing alternative treatments into a pain management strategy, it's important to do extensive study and speak with medical specialists since not all of them are supported by scientific data.

CHAPTER 7

Lifestyle Changes

Alcohol And Pancreatitis

Pancreatitis and alcohol have a complex interaction that must be understood to properly manage the illness. When the pancreas gets inflamed, it may cause pancreatitis, which manifests as a variety of symptoms including nausea, vomiting, and abdominal discomfort. Although alcoholism is not necessarily the cause of pancreatitis, it is a major risk factor, particularly when alcohol misuse is ongoing.

Although illness usually develops after years of excessive drinking, alcohol-induced pancreatitis may nevertheless strike anybody at any time. Although the precise processes by which alcohol causes pancreatitis are not entirely known, it is thought that alcohol may interfere with the pancreas' regular operation, causing inflammation and tissue damage to the organ.

Reducing or quitting alcohol is often an essential part of therapy and prevention for people with pancreatitis. Alcohol use, even in moderation, might worsen symptoms and raise the possibility of pancreatitis flare-ups. Consequently, leading a sober-focused lifestyle is crucial to properly treating the illness.

For those who are battling alcoholism, getting assistance from medical experts, support groups, or counseling services may be quite beneficial. These sites may provide direction, support, and techniques for staying sober and avoiding relapse.

Smoking Cessation

Another essential lifestyle modification for those with pancreatitis is quitting smoking. Similar to drinking, smoking increases the likelihood of developing pancreatitis and exacerbates its symptoms. Numerous dangerous compounds included in cigarette smoke may affect the pancreas and other organs, causing inflammation and raising the risk of pancreatitis.

Due to nicotine addiction, quitting smoking might be difficult, but it's an essential step in enhancing pancreatic health and general well-being. Thankfully, there are several tools and techniques available to assist in quitting smoking.

There are several methods available to those who want to stop smoking, including counseling, support groups, prescription medicine, and nicotine replacement therapy.

Furthermore, reducing cravings and increasing the likelihood of long-term success may be achieved by embracing better habits and discovering different coping mechanisms for stressful situations.

People with pancreatitis may greatly lower their chance of complications and enhance their quality of life by giving up smoking. During the quitting process, it is critical to have assistance from loved ones and medical specialists to optimize success and sustain motivation.

Exercise And Stress Management

In addition to being essential in controlling pancreatitis, regular exercise and stress reduction strategies also improve general health and well-being. Exercise benefits people with pancreatitis by lowering inflammation, promoting cardiovascular health, and helping people maintain a healthy weight.

Exercise must be done carefully, however, particularly when pancreatitis is recovering or flare-ups. Exercise may be beneficial without overtaxing the pancreas or aggravating symptoms if low-impact exercises like yoga, swimming, or walking are done.

Apart from physical activity, stress-reduction methods including progressive muscle relaxation, deep breathing exercises, and mindfulness meditation may enhance coping skills and lower stress levels. Effective stress management techniques are essential for the long-term treatment of pancreatitis since chronic stress has been related to inflammation and may worsen the condition's symptoms.

For those who have pancreatitis, finding pleasant hobbies and interests may also assist in lowering stress and enhancing overall quality of life. Making self-care and relaxation a priority may have a big impact on pancreatic health and general well-being, whether it's via relaxing, pursuing creative hobbies, or spending time with loved ones outside.

People with pancreatitis may take proactive measures to manage their illness and enhance their quality of life by adopting these lifestyle modifications into their everyday routines. A fulfilling and long-lasting aspect of living with pancreatitis may be forming healthy behaviors with commitment, assistance, and direction from medical specialists.

CHAPTER 8

Preventing Pancreatitis

Tips For Preventing Pancreatitis

It is important to prevent pancreatitis to preserve general health and well-being. The following useful advice can help you lower your chance of getting this condition:

1. Limit Alcohol intake: One of the main causes of pancreatitis is excessive alcohol intake. If you consume alcohol, do so sparingly. It is recommended that males have no more than two drinks each day, while women should only have one drink. Steer clear of excessive drinking since it greatly raises your risk of pancreatitis.

2. Maintain a Healthy Diet: For pancreatic health, a balanced diet is essential. Eat less fried and greasy meals since they might aggravate pancreatic inflammation. Rather, concentrate on eating an abundance of nutritious grains, fruits, veggies, and lean meats. Including foods high in antioxidants, such as spinach, berries, and almonds, may also aid in the reduction of inflammation.

3. Keep Yourself Hydrated: Avoiding pancreatitis requires consuming enough water. Be careful to stay hydrated throughout the day since dehydration might raise your chance of having this illness. Try to drink eight glasses of water or more if you exercise or spend time in hot conditions each day.

4. Give Up Smoking: Smoking raises your risk of pancreatitis in addition to being bad for your lungs. If you smoke, make an effort to stop as soon as you can. Giving up smoking may have a major positive impact on your general health and lower your chances of severe illnesses like pancreatitis.

5. Exercise Frequently: Physical exercise regularly is good for pancreatic health. Make an effort to engage in a minimum of 30 minutes of moderate activity on most days of the week. Exercises like swimming, cycling, or walking are great options. Your risk of pancreatitis may be decreased by exercising since it lowers inflammation, promotes general cardiovascular health, and helps you maintain a healthy weight.

6. Handle Chronic Conditions: Being obese, having diabetes, or having high cholesterol may all raise your chance of having pancreatitis. For these conditions to be properly managed, collaborate closely with your healthcare practitioner. To manage these illnesses and lower your risk of pancreatitis, adhere to their advice on medication, lifestyle modifications, and routine monitoring.

Healthy Habits For Pancreatic Health

Developing good habits is essential to maintaining the function of your pancreas and lowering your chance of developing pancreatitis. The following routines may be included in your everyday life to support pancreatic health:

1. **Eat a Balanced Diet:** Vital elements that promote pancreas function may be obtained by eating a diet high in fruits, vegetables, whole grains, and lean meats. Reducing the amount of fat and processed food consumed may help avoid pancreatic inflammation. Consume foods rich in antioxidants, such as almonds, leafy greens, and berries, to help fight inflammation and oxidative stress.

2. **Keep Yourself Hydrated:** Keeping your pancreas healthy requires proper hydration. By keeping pancreatic secretions from hardening, drinking enough water lowers the chance of obstructions

and inflammation. Try to consume eight glasses of water or more each day, and modify your amount according to the weather and degree of exercise.

3. Reduce Your Alcohol Consumption: Abuse of alcohol poses a serious risk for pancreatitis. Reducing or abstaining from alcohol may help shield the pancreas from harm and inflammation. If you decide to drink, make sure it's in moderation and don't overindulge. Women should keep to one drink each day, while males should restrict themselves to two.

4. Keep a Healthy Weight: Pancreatitis and other pancreatic problems are associated with obesity. Reaching and maintaining a healthy weight may be facilitated by adopting a healthy lifestyle that involves consistent exercise and eating a balanced diet. Make an effort to engage in a minimum of 30 minutes of moderate activity on most days of the week. You should also concentrate on eating wholesome meals in sensible portion amounts.

5. Give Up Smoking: Smoking raises the risk of pancreatic cancer and pancreatitis. One of the finest things you can do to safeguard the health of your pancreas is to stop smoking. To effectively stop smoking, enlist the help of friends, family, and medical experts. To assist control the symptoms of withdrawal, think about utilizing medicines or nicotine replacement therapy.

6. Handle Chronic illnesses: Pancreatic dysfunction and the risk of pancreatitis may be exacerbated by several chronic illnesses, including diabetes, obesity, and excessive cholesterol. For these conditions to be properly managed, collaborate closely with your healthcare practitioner. To keep these disorders under control and reduce their influence on pancreatic health, adhere to their suggestions for medication, lifestyle changes, and routine monitoring.

Importance Of Regular Check-Ups

To keep your pancreas healthy and identify any possible problems early, regular check-ups with your doctor are crucial. This is why routine examinations are so important:

1. **Early Problem Detection:** By monitoring your general health, your healthcare professional may identify any early indicators of inflammation or pancreatic malfunction. Early issue detection may prevent difficulties from developing and enhance the chance of a good outcome.

2. **Monitoring Chronic illnesses:** Routine examinations are necessary to monitor and evaluate the effects of any underlying chronic illnesses, such as diabetes or excessive cholesterol, on pancreatic health.

Your treatment plan might be modified by your healthcare practitioner as necessary to reduce the chance of problems like pancreatitis.

3. Assessment of Lifestyle variables: Your healthcare practitioner may talk to you about lifestyle variables, such as food, alcohol usage, and smoking, during checkups. These factors may have an impact on pancreatic health. They can give you tools and assistance to help you make healthy lifestyle choices, as well as advice on how to make them.

4. Pancreatic cancer screening: Although less prevalent than other pancreatic illnesses, pancreatic cancer is a dangerous and often fatal illness. Screenings and conversations on your risk factors for pancreatic cancer may be part of your routine check-ups. The prognosis for pancreatic cancer is better with early diagnosis, leading to longer life and more effective therapy.

5. Building a Relationship with Your Provider: By seeing your doctor regularly, you may build a trustworthy rapport with them. Open communication is facilitated by this connection, which makes it simpler to voice worries, pose inquiries, and look for advice on preserving pancreatic health.

6. Preventive Measures: Vaccinations and screens for other medical issues are examples of preventive measures that may be included in routine check-ups, in addition to monitoring your present health state. Pancreatic health may be indirectly supported and the risk of pancreatitis and other pancreatic illnesses can be decreased by taking proactive measures to preserve general health.

You may prevent pancreatitis and other pancreatic problems by proactively maintaining pancreatic health and collaborating closely with your healthcare professional.

CHAPTER 9

Living With Pancreatitis

Support Systems And Resources

Living with pancreatitis may be difficult, but managing the illness can be greatly improved by having a solid support network and easy access to useful information. Creating a network of friends, family, medical experts, and support groups may provide informational support, practical help, and emotional support.

Particularly during flare-ups or hospital stays, family and friends are invaluable in assisting with everyday chores and offering emotional support. They may provide support, listen, help with housework, or provide transportation to doctor's appointments. It is possible to build stronger bonds and promote understanding by being open and honest with loved ones about your needs, fears, and conditions.

Medical experts such as physicians, nurses, nutritionists, and therapists are vital in the management of pancreatitis. In addition to monitoring your health and prescribing drugs, they may give medical advice and make nutritional suggestions based on your requirements. Establishing a rapport of trust with your medical team facilitates efficient communication and cooperative decision-making, guaranteeing that you get the finest treatment possible.

People with pancreatitis may find understanding and a feeling of camaraderie via attending in-person or virtual support groups. Making connections with others who have gone through similar things to you may provide support, understanding, and useful coping mechanisms. Through information sharing, emotional support, and encouragement from one another, support group meetings, forums, and social media platforms enable people with pancreatitis to manage their condition more skillfully.

Furthermore, there are several tools accessible to inform and support those who have pancreatitis. Education regarding the illness, available treatments, self-care techniques, and lifestyle adjustments may be found on websites, online forums, and educational materials. Having access to trustworthy information sources helps people make choices about their health and well-being, which improves their capacity to successfully manage pancreatitis.

Pancreatitis patients may improve their quality of life, lower their stress levels, and more effectively manage the difficulties that come with their disease by developing a strong support system and making use of the tools that are readily accessible to them. The experience of living with pancreatitis may be greatly enhanced by using support networks and services, whether one is looking for practical help, emotional support, or insightful knowledge.

Psychological Impact Of Pancreatitis

In addition to its medical effects, pancreatitis has a significant psychological influence on those who have it. Reducing the quality of life and causing mental anguish, worry, and depression are some of the consequences of controlling symptoms, following dietary restrictions, and coping with chronic pain.

Pancreatitis often manifests as chronic pain, which may significantly affect mental health. Sustaining pain may hurt mood, sleep, day-to-day activities, and general quality of life. It can also cause emotions of despair, helplessness, and frustration. Effective pain management calls for a multifaceted strategy that takes into account psychological as well as physical factors. This includes prescription drugs, mindfulness exercises, relaxation methods, and psychological therapies.

Taking care of symptoms including nausea, vomiting, exhaustion, and digestive issues in addition to pain management will help with psychological difficulties and emotional anguish. These symptoms may cause feelings of loneliness, annoyance, and loss of independence by interfering with day-to-day activities, social contacts, and work. By learning symptom management methods, creating coping mechanisms, and getting assistance from medical experts, people may deal with these difficulties more skillfully.

Another feature of pancreatitis that may affect psychological health is dietary limitations. A pancreatitis-friendly diet often entails staying away from foods and drinks that may aggravate inflammation or cause symptoms. This dietary strategy may include big adjustments to food preparation, social engagement, and eating habits, which may be emotionally taxing and alienating from others. Getting assistance from friends, investigating substitute foods and cooking techniques, and seeing a nutritionist may all help people follow dietary guidelines more closely and feel more satisfied with their meal selections overall.

Furthermore, having pancreatitis may lead to uncertainty about the future due to worries about how the condition will proceed, possible complications, how treatment will work, and the prognosis in the long run. Being uncertain may exacerbate feelings of worry, anxiety, and dread of the unknown, which makes it challenging to be optimistic and make plans for the future. others may learn to manage uncertainty and reclaim control over their life by talking openly with healthcare practitioners, learning as much as they can about the disease, and making connections with like-minded others.

A comprehensive strategy that incorporates medical treatment, psychological assistance, self-care techniques, and social support is necessary to address the psychosocial effects of pancreatitis. People may strengthen their coping mechanisms, develop resilience in the face of hardship, and improve their mental health by recognizing and treating the emotional difficulties connected to the illness.

Maintaining Quality Of Life

Living with pancreatitis requires a proactive strategy that takes care of the practical, social, emotional, and physical components of well-being to maintain a good quality of life.

Notwithstanding the difficulties the illness presents, there are several tactics people may use to improve their general quality of life and foster happiness and wellness.

Maintaining quality of life in the face of pancreatitis requires good symptom management. This includes taking prescription drugs as directed, eating healthily, managing stress, and getting help right away if there are problems or flare-ups in the body. Through quick and proactive symptom management, people may reduce pain, enhance function, and maximize their overall state of health.

For those who have pancreatitis, frequent physical exercise may help improve their quality of life. Exercise has been shown to increase mood, lower stress levels, increase physical fitness and support general health and wellbeing. Including exercise routines like yoga, tai chi, walking, or swimming may have several advantages, such as better symptom management, more energy, and better sleep.

Maintaining one's quality of life while dealing with pancreatitis also requires giving priority to one's mental and emotional well-being. This might include getting help from mental health specialists, going to therapy or counseling, doing deep breathing exercises or meditation, and developing an optimistic view of life. People may live more satisfying and fulfilled lives and more effectively manage the difficulties of having a chronic illness by attending to their emotional needs and developing resilience.

A person's quality of life is greatly impacted by social support while they have pancreatitis. During trying times, reaching out to friends, family, support groups, and medical experts may provide consolation, empathy, and useful help. Developing and maintaining supportive connections may improve general well-being, provide a sense of belonging, and lessen feelings of loneliness.

Participating in joyful, fulfilling, and meaningful activities may also enhance one's quality of life. Whether it's via volunteering, engaging in new activities, hobbies, or time spent with loved ones, finding moments of pleasure and purpose may strengthen resilience and raise general life satisfaction.

In general, preserving quality of life in the face of pancreatitis requires a comprehensive strategy that takes into account practical, social, emotional, and physical demands. People with pancreatitis may maximize their quality of life and lead fulfilling lives by taking proactive measures to manage their symptoms, giving self-care priority, getting assistance, and engaging in activities that enhance well-being.

CHAPTER 10

Future Directions

Research And Innovations In Pancreatitis

Understanding the shifting environment of scientific investigation and medical developments is vital as we explore into the future of pancreatitis research and innovations. To enhance patient diagnosis, care, and quality of life, researchers from all over the world are devoting their lives to understanding the complexity of pancreatitis.

Determining the fundamental causes of pancreatitis is an intriguing field of study. Researchers are focusing on the molecular processes, hereditary inclinations, and environmental elements that influence the onset and course of this illness. Novel therapeutic targets may be found by comprehending these subtleties, opening the door to more potent therapies.

In addition, pancreatitis diagnosis and surveillance are being revolutionized by advances in imaging methods. Unmatched insights into pancreatic shape and function are provided by high-resolution imaging modalities such as endoscopic ultrasound (EUS) and magnetic resonance imaging (MRI). With the use of these non-invasive techniques, medical professionals may identify minute alterations in the pancreas early on, allowing for prompt intervention and better patient outcomes.

When it comes to pancreatitis therapy, tailored medicine is starting to show promise. With the use of molecular diagnostics and genetic profiling, medical professionals may customize treatment plans for each patient, increasing effectiveness and reducing side effects. Furthermore, individuals with significant damage may be able to regain pancreatic function thanks to regenerative therapy, which offers hope for a long-term recovery.

Another factor promoting innovation in pancreatitis research is cooperation between academic institutions, businesses, and medical professionals. To address this complex illness from all fronts, interdisciplinary teams are combining their knowledge, which promotes a synergistic strategy that advances treatment faster. Additionally, programs like clinical trial networks and open-access data repositories are making it easier for people to collaborate and share data globally, which is hastening the application of research results in the clinic.

The field of pancreatitis research is full of opportunities as we move to the future. With unwavering commitment, creativity, and teamwork, we can strive to revolutionize the way this illness is treated, providing millions of people with hope and recovery throughout the globe.

Promising Treatments On The Horizon

Numerous new approaches that have the potential to transform patient care are shining light on the pancreatitis treatment future. The range of therapeutic choices is growing, from less invasive surgeries to innovative pharmacotherapies, providing hope to those struggling with this difficult ailment.

Pharmacological drugs that target certain molecular pathways involved in the pathophysiology of pancreatitis represent one area of investigation. These include substances that promote pancreatic regeneration, modulators of pancreatic enzyme output, and inhibitors of inflammatory cytokines. These drugs can act at the molecular level to reduce inflammation, relieve symptoms, and encourage tissue healing, opening up new possibilities for the treatment of diseases.

Minimally invasive treatments are becoming more and more popular as effective treatment choices for pancreatitis, in addition to medication. With the ability to precisely administer medications straight to the pancreas, endoscopic procedures like endoscopic retrograde cholangiopancreatography (ERCP) and endoscopic ultrasonography (EUS) are being used more and more for therapeutic reasons. These techniques, which range from endoscopic necrosectomy to pseudocyst drainage, provide less intrusive substitutes for conventional surgery while lowering morbidity and speeding healing.

Moreover, the range of pancreatitis therapy alternatives is growing because of developments in interventional radiology. Fluid accumulation and vascular problems may be effectively managed with the use of techniques like percutaneous drainage and pseudoaneurysm embolization. Through the use of image-guided therapies, healthcare professionals may precisely target pathology, hence improving patient outcomes.

Regenerative medicine has great potential to treat pancreatitis in addition to traditional therapy. New methods for repairing tissue damage and regaining pancreatic function include stem cell treatment, tissue engineering, and gene editing technologies. These innovative treatments seek to revolutionize pancreatitis care by using the body's regenerative potential to provide hope for sustained remission and enhanced quality of life.

The prognosis for pancreatitis care is improving as these effective therapies go through thorough assessment and clinical trials. For those impacted by this complicated illness, we can usher in a new age of individualized, efficient, and compassionate treatment by embracing innovation, teamwork, and a patient-centered approach.

Advocacy And Awareness Efforts

The battle against pancreatitis must include advocacy and awareness since they are essential in bringing about change, giving patients and their families a sense of empowerment, and providing support. Advocacy initiatives seek to improve outcomes and quality of life for those impacted by pancreatitis by increasing knowledge of the warning signs, symptoms, and risk factors connected to the condition.

Raising awareness of the frequency and consequences of this often disregarded illness among the general public and medical professionals is one of the main goals of pancreatitis advocacy. Through debunking myths and promoting a better knowledge of pancreatitis, advocacy groups enable people to seek prompt medical treatment and get the right therapy. Additionally, via interacting with legislators, medical professionals, and the media, advocates may push for better access to treatment, more money for research, and better support services for pancreatitis sufferers and their families.

Moreover, advocacy initiatives are essential in de-stigmatizing pancreatitis and lessening the stigma and loneliness that many patients endure. Advocacy groups help those impacted by pancreatitis feel a sense of community, belonging, and solidarity by encouraging self-sufficiency, optimism, and empowerment via peer support, story-sharing, and event planning.

Advocacy groups are essential for supporting patients and their families by offering information and assistance in addition to campaigning for governmental changes and increasing public awareness. These organizations provide financial aid programs, educational events, online support groups, and instructional resources that help people overcome the problems of pancreatitis. They also give counsel, encouragement, and practical assistance at every step of the process.

In the next years, advocacy and awareness campaigns will be crucial for advancing research, encouraging teamwork, and improving the prognosis of pancreatitis patients. We can bring about significant change and guarantee that all individuals affected by this illness get the attention, assistance, and compassion they are entitled to by elevating the voices of patients, caregivers, and healthcare professionals.

CONCLUSION

Pancreatitis requires quick diagnosis and effective care due to its complexity and potential for life-threatening consequences. We have examined the causes, signs, diagnosis, and available treatments for pancreatitis throughout this investigation, emphasizing the multifaceted character of the condition and the value of individualized patient care.

First, we went over the main causes of pancreatitis, which include alcohol intake, gallstones, genetics, and certain drugs. It is essential to comprehend these triggers to prevent pancreatitis from developing in the first place and to design successful treatment plans.

Second, the signs and symptoms of pancreatitis, which range from nausea and stomach discomfort to more serious issues including organ failure, highlight how important it is to identify the disease early and take appropriate action. Early diagnosis with blood testing and imaging methods may greatly enhance patient outcomes.

Thirdly, the course of therapy for pancreatitis varies according to its severity and underlying cause. While less severe bouts may merely need supportive treatment and pain control, more severe instances may require hospitalization, fluid resuscitation, and possibly surgery to address complications such as pseudocysts or necrosis.

Additionally, we've looked at how lifestyle adjustments including diet adjustments and alcohol abstinence might help manage chronic pancreatitis and stop repeated attacks. The key to long-term care and lowering the risk of problems is patient education and adherence to recommended regimens.

Pancreatitis, which requires a thorough knowledge of its origin, symptomatology, and treatment choices, essentially represents the junction of medical science and patient care. Healthcare practitioners may work toward better results and an enhanced quality of life for those impacted by this difficult illness by using developments in diagnostic technology, treatment modalities, and holistic patient management techniques. To better understand the complexity of pancreatitis and improve our approaches to its treatment and prevention, ongoing study and cooperation are crucial.

THE END